AN INTRODUCTION TO

MOTIF NOTATION

AN INTRODUCTION TO

MOTIF NOTATION

by

Ann Hutchinson Guest

Language of Dance Centre

Published by:
Language of Dance Centre
17 Holland Park
London
W11 5DT
United Kingdom

Distributed by:
Dance Books Ltd.
The Old Bakery
4 Lenten Street
Alton,
Hampshire, GU34 1HG
United Kingdom

First publication 2007

Nielsen Book Data

Dr. Hutchinson Guest, Ann
      An Introduction to Motif Notation.
      1. A/AS Level,
      2. Adult Education,
      3. Further/higher Education,
      4. Professionally and scholarly

ISBN 978-0-9554305-0-3

TABLE OF CONTENTS

INTRODUCTION

The purpose of this book is to provide a simple introduction to Motif Notation as used in the Language of Dance® movement exploration. The presentation of the material is designed to provide an easy transition into the more detailed usage of Motif presented in *Your Move – The Language of Dance Approach to the Study of Movement and Dance.*

Introduction to Motif Notation has intentionally been kept brief, with the knowledge that further information is available.

An in-depth study of Language of Dance requires time, but use of the Motif symbols can begin at an elementary level and be applied as needed in each situation. It is anticipated that this book will be a welcome guide for those becoming interested in using Motif Notation. Note that Motif Notation is also called Motif Writing. Some do still refer to it as Motif Writing as well as Motif Description.

First published in 1983, *Your Move* has been extensively used by students and teachers, demonstrating a greater need for clarification in both movement understanding and in use of the symbols. The particular value of *Your Move* is the depth of movement analysis that it provides and the understanding of what the Motif symbols represent.

I wish to acknowledge the helpful comments on this book contributed by Anne Green Gilbert, Susan Gingrasso and Tina Curran who made valuable suggestions on text clarification. For the preparation of this book for publication, my thanks and great appreciation go to the staff at the Language of Dance Centre, Lynda Howarth, Carolyn Griffiths, and in particular Silke Wiegand who contributed to the layout of the pages as well as the task of producing the Motif symbols with the Calaban computer program.

Ann Hutchinson Guest

MOTIF HISTORY

Motif Notation, also known as Motif Description and Motif Writing, is one system for graphically representing and recording movement; it is closely related to Labanotation. These two systems use most of the same symbols and terminology, have a similar format, and both record fundamental components, such as direction, action, dynamics, relationship and timing, that are found in all styles and forms of movement.

Ann Hutchinson Guest, the outstanding developer of Rudolf Laban's system of Kinetography for which she coined the name "Labanotation", began to explore using the notation symbols in a freer, more exploratory way while teaching children at the New York City 92nd Street Y.M.H.A. in the 1950s. It was this experience which inspired her to identify the list of prime movement actions universal to all movement forms. After research, which included consulting many lists and sources such as the 'Seven Movements in Dance', as taught in the Cecchetti Classical Ballet Method, Laban's list of basic actions and the writings of Margart H'Doubler, she codified what she felt to be the ABC's of movement, now termed the Movement Alphabet®.

In England, the need for a freer use of the Labanotation symbols arose when Valerie Preston Dunlop was teaching Laban's Educational Dance to physical education teachers. It was one of these teachers who suggested the very appropriate name, Motif Writing. This led to Valerie's development of the usage, and to the subsequent publication in 1967 of her books on the subject entitled *Readers in Kinetography Laban, Series B, Motif Writing for Dance*.

In 1971, while teaching movement analysis and notation at the Teacher Training College of the Royal Academy of Dancing, Guest further developed her exploratory and creative use of the Motif symbols. She recognized the need for complex movements to be deconstructed to their most basic elements with focus on the key elements. It was during this time that she codified the Language of Dance® work and produced the textbook entitled *Your Move - A New Approach to the Study of Movement and Dance* published in 1983.

Motif is used internationally in diverse contexts and with different approaches and applications. The use of Motif provides an accessible link to movement for participants of all ages and skill levels; it is applicable to any technique, style or genre of dance or other movement forms. Motif provides an easy introduction to dance literacy through the visual symbols and clear movement vocabulary.

THE MOVEMENT ALPHABET® - THE VERBS

The prime actions and concepts of which movement is comprised are as follows:

Presence or Absence of Movement

Intitial Statements

| 1. | | **Any Action** | Movement of some kind, a change |
| 2. | | **Stillness** | Suspension of motion, sustainment of an arrested activity |

An action may be concerned with or may focus on

Anatomical Possibilities

3.		**Flexion**	Contracting, folding, closing in, making smaller, narrowing
4.		**Extension**	Lengthening, reaching out, enlarging, opening out, elongating, unfolding
5.		**Rotation**	Any revolution, rotation of the body-as-a-whole, or of parts of the body

Spatial Aspects

| 6. | | **Traveling** | Any path (straight, circular, meandering or curving) moving from one place to another |
| 7. | | **Direction** | Movement into different directions such as up, down, to the right, left, forward, backward |

Supporting

| 8. | | **Support** | An action ending in a new support, transference of weight |
| 9. | | **A Spring** | Any aerial step; leaving the ground and returning to it |

Center of Gravity

| 10. | | **Balance** | Equilibrium, centre of weight vertically over a moving or static support |
| 11. | | **Falling** | Not in balance: centre of weight moves beyond point of support; loss of balance results. |

Motion, Destination

Movement Intention

12.		**Motion Toward**	Approaching a person, object, direction, or state; a gesture toward oneself
13.		**Motion Away**	Leaving, withdrawing from a person, object, direction, or state; a gesture away from oneself
14.		**Destination**	Statement of an ending situation, position or state to be reached

- -

RESULTS   ◇   **Any still shape**   **Any form of relating**

GENERAL STATEMENT

AN ACTION, ANY ACTION

The most basic instruction to move is shown by a vertical line,
1a. When something quite out of context is needed, the added
freedom of 'any', can be given, 1b. The sign for 'any' can be
drawn horizontally or vertically, 1c, 1d.

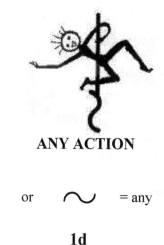

ANY ACTION

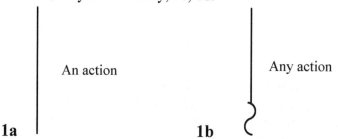

1a An action   **1b** Any action   **1c** or ∼ = any   **1d**

Duration

The amount of time taken to perform the movement is shown by the length of the action stroke. Note
the double horizontal line to indicate the start of movement, the movement is read up the page. A very
slight gap between action strokes shows that they are two separate symbols.

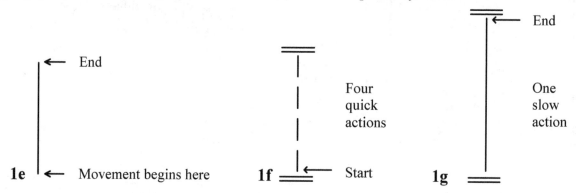

1e ← End   ← Movement begins here   **1f** ← Start   Four quick actions   **1g** One slow action   ← End

Length of Pause, Gap

The definite space between the action strokes shows a moment of inactivity. In 1h the two quick
actions are followed by a pause of some duration. Two quick actions occur again. These may be quite
different actions from the first two.

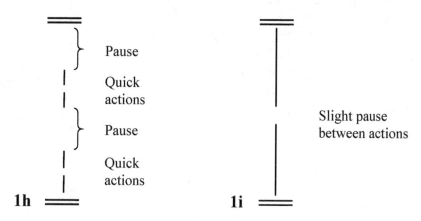

1h Pause / Quick actions / Pause / Quick actions   **1i** Slight pause between actions

1

STILLNESS

When no movement is indicated, the position arrived at may be actively held, as in playing statues, or the energy, the expression can continue, in a way comparable to the resonance of sound in music when it is not suddenly cut off. Holding, retaining a position is shown by a small circle, 2a. If the position is to be alive, continue to have breath, to be ready for what will soon follow, then the V sign of 1b is added to the hold sign, producing 2c.

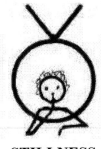

STILLNESS

2a ◯ = Hold   **2b** ∨ = Energy outflowing   **2c** ◯̌ = Stillness

The gap between the action strokes (the movement indications) in 2d means no action, no change, i.e. the absence of movement. During this gap, the performer may intentionally hold the end result of the previous movement, the position of arrival, as indicated by the hold sign in 2e, or the quality, expression of the previous movement may continue so that the gap is filled with stillness, 2f. Note that the gap together with the symbol indicates the duration of the stillness or of the holding.

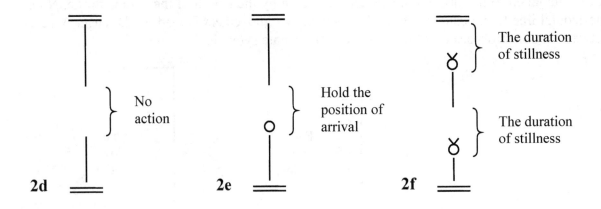

2d — No action   2e — Hold the position of arrival   2f — The duration of stillness / The duration of stillness

Holding a Position

Static holding during a pause, a gap, may be intended as a shape, that is, ending in an interesting position, similar to the children's game of "statues". Example 2g is the sign for "a shape". An action stroke, indicating how long it takes to arrive in that position, is linked to the sign for shape with a small vertical bow. The hold sign and the gap that follows indicate how long the position is held, 2h.

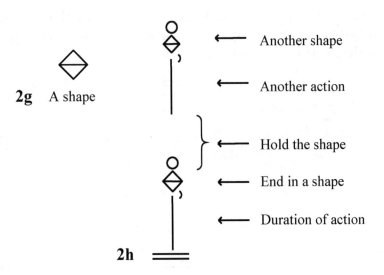

2g A shape

← Another shape

← Another action

← Hold the shape

← End in a shape

← Duration of action

2h

2

MEASURED TIME

So far, only a general indication of time – quick or slow - has been given. The first step in organizing time is to indicate a span of time. This is shown between double horizontal lines, 3a. Next, measures of time are placed between horizontal bar lines, comparable to music bar lines. Ex. 3b shows three measures of time. In 3c the meter of 3/4 is stated, i.e. 3 quarter notes in each measure. The end of each beat (count) and the start of the next are shown by a small tick mark.

Span of Time

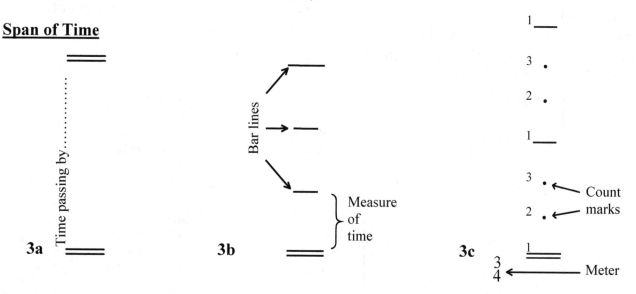

Numbers for the counts are written small while the numbering of each measure is shown with larger numbers. Ex. 3d shows 4 measures of 2/4, while 3e gives 2 measures of 4/4.

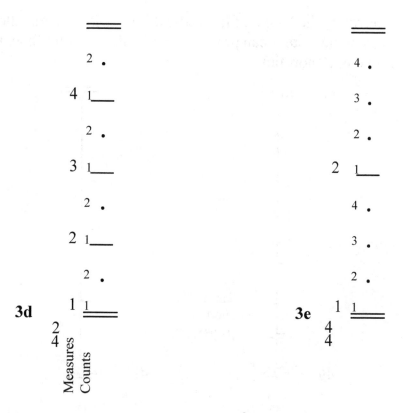

3

SPATIAL ASPECTS

TRAVELLING

Travelling is a familiar activity, but what form does the resulting path take? It may be straight, curving or circular. For first explorations freedom is given in allowing 'any path' to be chosen. 'Any path' is shown by horizontal ad lib. signs placed at both ends of an action stroke, 4a. Ex. 4b shows a straight path, while 4c is a curving path. A circular path is shown by slanting lines. Ex. 4d shows circling counter clockwise (CCW) while 4e states circling clockwise (CW). When the direction of circling is to be open to choice, the composite sign of 4f is used.

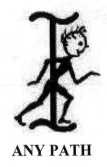

ANY PATH

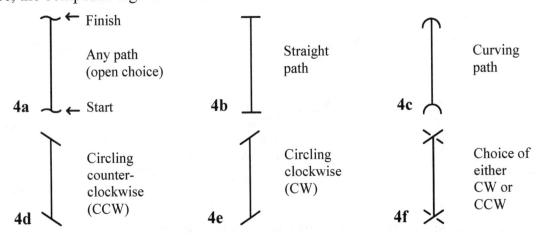

Duration of Path (Travelling)

The duration of the path is shown by the length of the vertical line. Distance travelled is often linked to duration. A few steps or slow steps can produce a path taking longer time, whereas running can cover much ground in a short time.

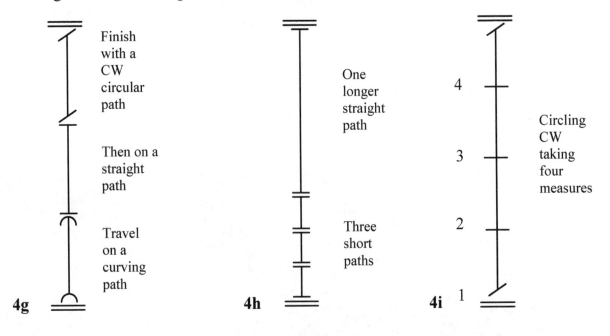

FLOOR PLANS

A floor plan 'map' is helpful in showing how the room (stage area) is being used. The open rectangle of 5a shows the room, the open part being the front where the audience is. Pins are used to indicate the performer on the stage. A white pin, 5b, represents a woman, a black pin, 5c, a man and the straight 'tack', 6d shows a person with no indication of gender.

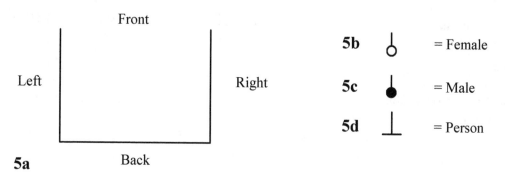

Placement on the stage area shows where the dancers are located. The point of the pin indicates the direction to which the performers are facing.

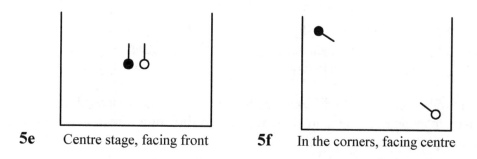

Each plan should start where the previous one ended. Note the following sequence:

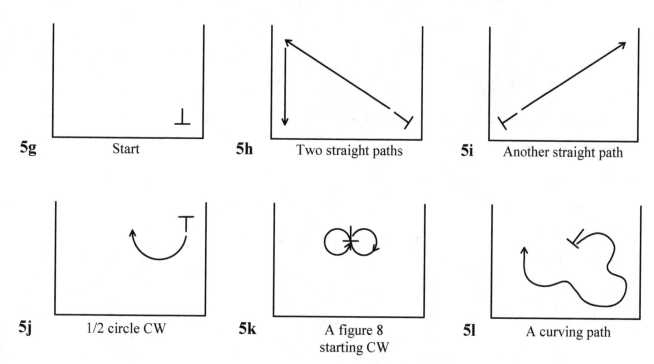

DIRECTIONS FOR TRAVELLING

Choice of direction may be left open. The rectangle of 6a is the basic sign for direction. Freedom in choice of direction is shown in 6b.

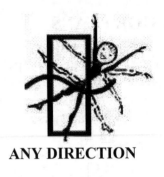

ANY DIRECTION

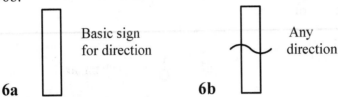

In 6c and 6d no step direction is stated, it is open to choice. Ex. 6e shows the more direct statement of 'any direction' for the straight path.

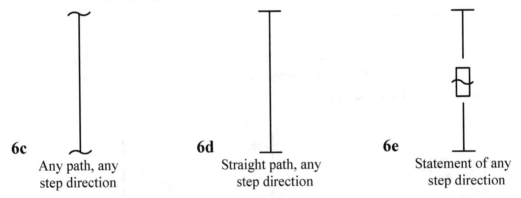

From a starting place, travelling can be into different directions – forward, backward, to the right or to the left. The shape of the rectangle is changed to show the chosen direction: forward, 6f, backward, 6g, to the left, 6h, and to the right 6i.

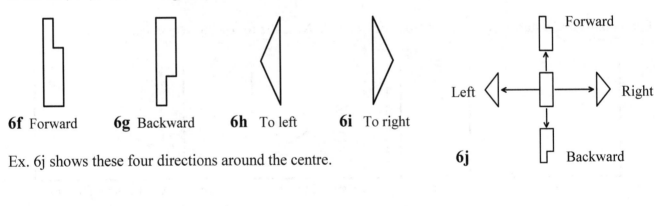

Ex. 6j shows these four directions around the centre.

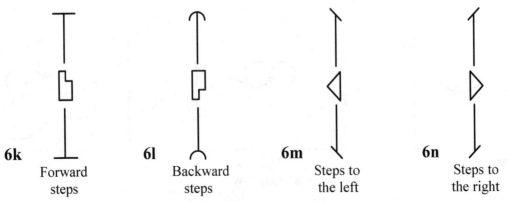

6

DIRECTION FOR CIRCULAR PATH

Circular paths with forward steps have the centre of the circle at the performer's right when circling CW, 7a, and at the left when circling CCW, 7b. Backward steps while circling CCW has the centre of the circle at the right, 7c, and at the left when circling CW with backward steps, 7d.

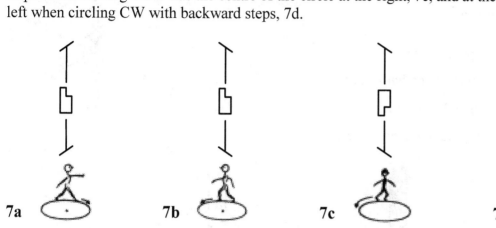

The performer faces to the centre of the circle when taking sideward steps are to the right and circling is CCW, 7e. When sideward steps to the left are taken, circling is CW, 7f. The performer's back is to the centre of the circle when circling CW with steps to the right, 7g, and also when steps are to the left and circling is CCW, 7h.

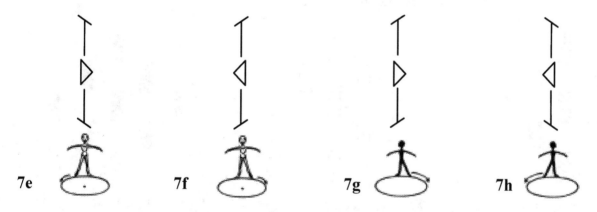

The following floor plans can help in visualizing such circling. The men in 7i are all facing CW, they may travel forward (CW) or backward (CCW) when in this arrangement. The women in 7j are all facing in, thus steps to the right will make them travel CCW, and steps to the left will produce CW circling. Facing out, as in 7k, produces the reverse, steps to the right travel CW, to the left will travel CCW.

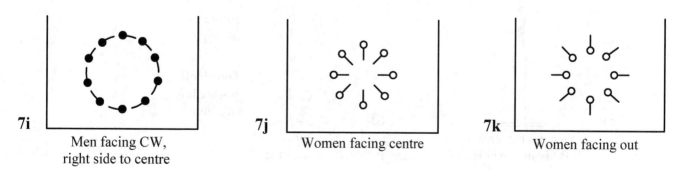

7i — Men facing CW, right side to centre

7j — Women facing centre

7k — Women facing out

DIRECTIONS FOR GESTURES

The dimensional directions around the body can be combined with level – high, horizontal (middle), and low – to produce the 27 main directions.

The Dimensional Directions

In the vertical dimension – up and down

In the sagittal dimension – forward and backward

In the lateral dimension – left and right sides

The shading of the direction symbol indicates the level:

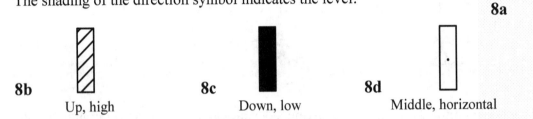

8b Up, high

8c Down, low

8d Middle, horizontal

Each of the directions can be in a high level, a low level or a middle level.

The 27 Main Directions

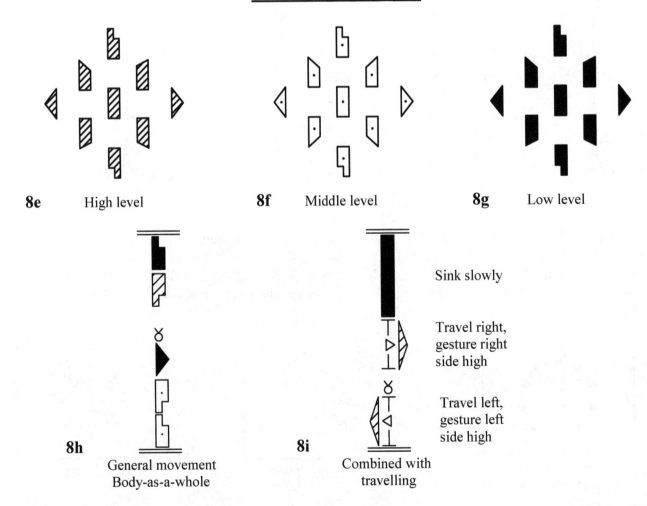

8e High level

8f Middle level

8g Low level

8h General movement
Body-as-a-whole

8i Combined with
travelling

Sink slowly

Travel right,
gesture right
side high

Travel left,
gesture left
side high

ANATOMICAL POSSIBILITIES

ROTATION, TURNING

Rotations of the whole body may be pivot turns, somersaults or cartwheels. Ex. 9a is the sign giving open choice for any kind of rotation. First we will deal with the most familiar form, rotation around the vertical axis. Ex 9b shows turning to the left, while 9c is turning to the right. The choice of pivoting either way is shown by the composite sign of 9d.

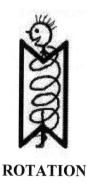

ROTATION

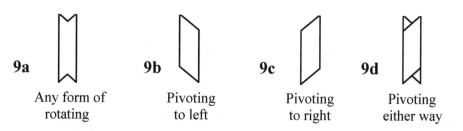

9a	9b	9c	9d
Any form of rotating	Pivoting to left	Pivoting to right	Pivoting either way

Degree of Turning, Circling

Turning often occurs to face into another room direction. Such turning establishes a new Front, a new orientation to the room (stage) directions. The degree of turning is shown by a black pin inside the turn sign. These degrees are also applied to the pathway signs for circling.

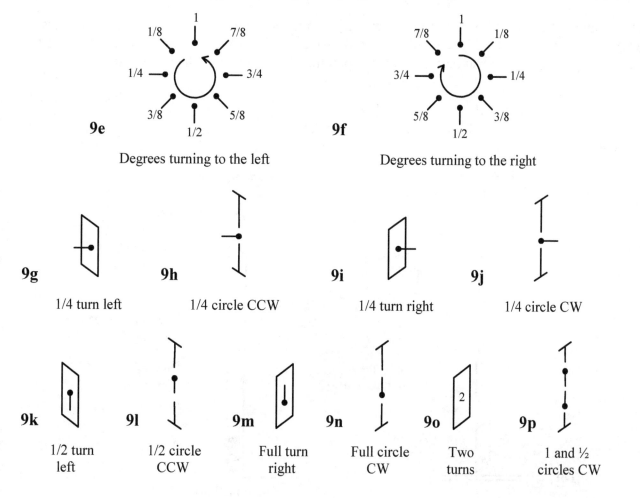

9e — Degrees turning to the left

9f — Degrees turning to the right

9g — 1/4 turn left

9h — 1/4 circle CCW

9i — 1/4 turn right

9j — 1/4 circle CW

9k — 1/2 turn left

9l — 1/2 circle CCW

9m — Full turn right

9n — Full circle CW

9o — Two turns

9p — 1 and ½ circles CW

9

Other Forms: Twist, Somersault, Cartwheel

Twist

The signs for pivot turns, 10a, that is, rotations around the vertical axis, can be applied to turns, rotations of the torso and limbs. While the whole body can rotate completely in one piece, the torso and limbs are attached and hence the free end can turn to a greater degree than the part closer to the base, thus producing a twist. To show this twist, a hold sign is placed at the base of the turn sign, 10b-c.

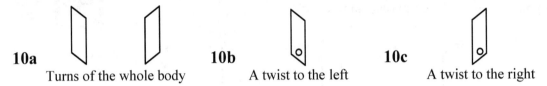

10a   Turns of the whole body   **10b**   A twist to the left   **10c**   A twist to the right

Somersault

The statement 'any form of rotation', 10d, could be a somersault forward, 10e, or backward, 10f.

10d = Any rotation   **10e** = Forward somersault   **10f** = Backward somersault

Cartwheel

Equally, 'any rotation' could be a cartwheel revolution to the left, 10g, or to the right, 10h. Because a full cartwheel incorporates a hidden full turn (full change of Front), an ordinary turn sign is at the centre of the symbol. At top and bottom, 'arrows' pointing the direction of the cartwheel are added.

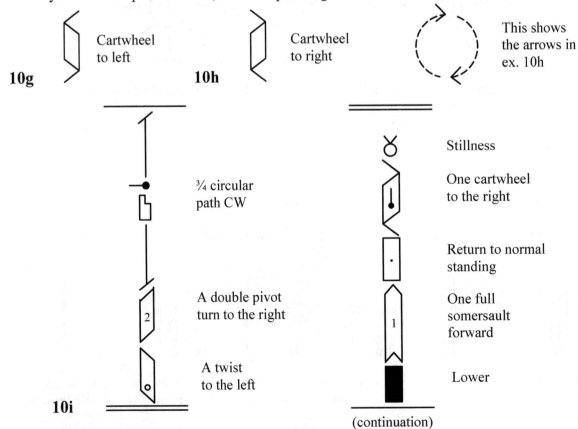

10g Cartwheel to left   **10h** Cartwheel to right   This shows the arrows in ex. 10h

¾ circular path CW

A double pivot turn to the right

A twist to the left

10i

Stillness

One cartwheel to the right

Return to normal standing

One full somersault forward

Lower

(continuation)

ORIENTATION

To establish where you are facing in the room, the Front Signs are used. After each turn a new Front Sign is shown. Once the Front is established in the room it remains constant.

The Front Signs

11a

After a turn, the new Front sign is placed at the left of the movement indications.

11b Facing Front (audience)

11c Back to audience

11d In profile, face stage left

11e In profile, face stage right

11f Left front diagonal

11g Right front diagonal

11h Left back diagonal

11i Right back diagonal

Note the Front indications in the following sequences: Ex. 11j produces a square; 11k travels on a straight line; 11l retraces the half circular path.

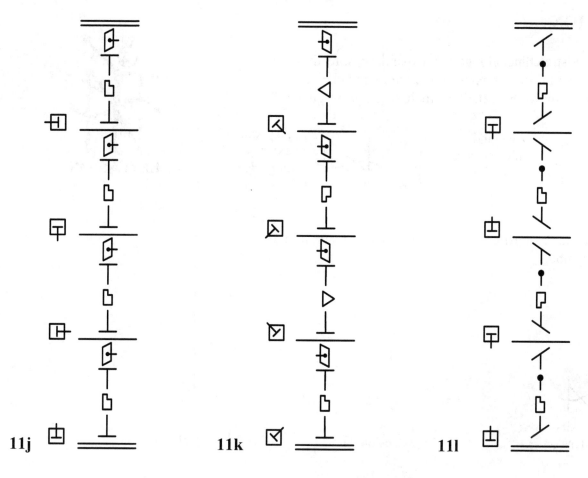

11j   11k   11l

FLEXION

Drawing in, contracting, folding, curling up etc. are all forms of flexion. Freedom in the choice of which form to use is shown by 12a, the sign for 'any flexion'. Two main degrees are given:

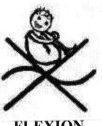

FLEXION

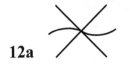 **12a** — Any kind of flexion, small degree

12b 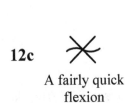 — Any kind of flexion, large degree

Duration of flexing is shown by the addition of an attached duration line.

12c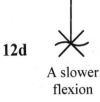
A fairly quick flexion

12d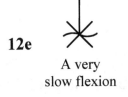
A slower flexion

12e
A very slow flexion

EXTENSION

Reaching out, stretching, elongating, expanding, spreading, abducting, are all forms of extension. Freedom in choice of which to use if shown by 12f. Two main degrees are given:

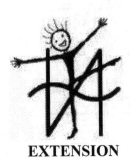

EXTENSION

12f 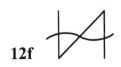 — Any kind of extension, small degree

12g 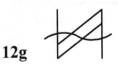 — Any kind of extension, large degree

Duration of such extension is shown by attaching a duration line to the symbol.

12h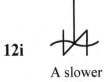
Any kind of extension

12i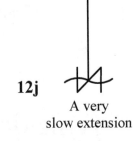
A slower extension

12j
A very slow extension

RETAIN, CANCEL

A state produced by a movement, for instance an extended state, may need to be held, retained while another movement occurs. A stated retention must, at some point, be cancelled. Ex. 13a is the sign for holding or retaining. The narrow inverted V is the sign for cancellation, 13b, it has the meaning "no longer in effect."

13a ◯ = Retain   **13b** ∧ = Cancel; the previous is no longer in effect

In the following reading examples such retention and cancellation are shown.

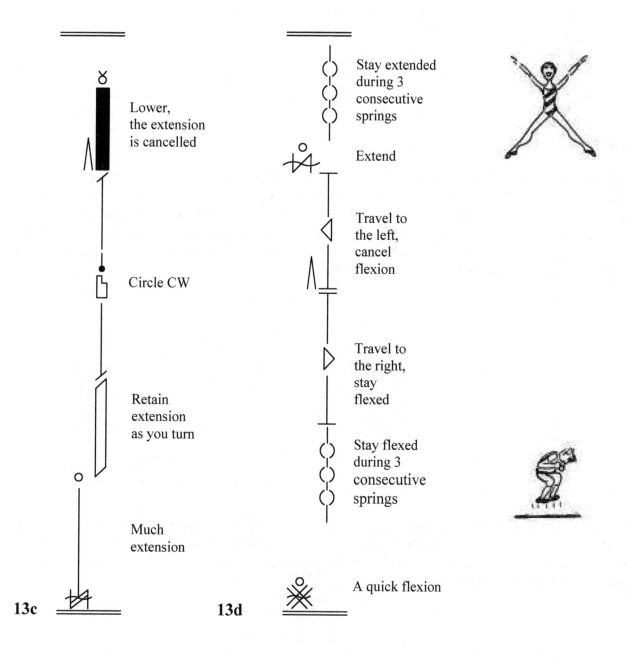

Lower, the extension is cancelled

Circle CW

Retain extension as you turn

Much extension

13c

Stay extended during 3 consecutive springs

Extend

Travel to the left, cancel flexion

Travel to the right, stay flexed

Stay flexed during 3 consecutive springs

A quick flexion

13d

SPECIFIC FORMS OF FLEXION AND EXTENSION

Contracting, Elongating

Contracting is the form of flexion in which the extremity of the limb draws in toward the body (toward its base) on a straight line. As a result, the centre joint, the elbow in the case of the arm, will be displaced in space. In 14a, 'Z' marks the extremity and 'X' the base, with 'Y' the mid joint. With multi-jointed parts, the hand and the spine, the centre part bulges out on a curve, 14b. The symbol for contraction is 14c with 14d the greater amount. Elongating is the reverse of contracting, the extremity extends on a straight line. Only one degree of elongation is usually needed, 14e.

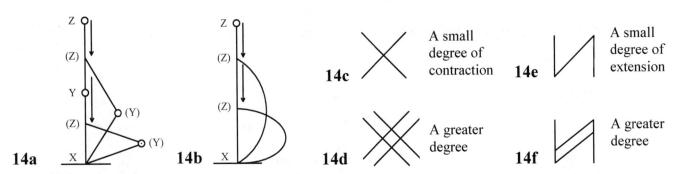

14a

14b

14c — A small degree of contraction

14d — A greater degree

14e — A small degree of extension

14f — A greater degree

Folding, Unfolding

Folding is the form of flexion in which the limb extremity closes in toward its base on a curved path. Ex. 15a illustrates the folding in of the extremity 'C' toward the base 'A'. Ex. 15b is the basic sign for folding over any body surface, the horizontal ad lib. sign indicating this freedom of choice. Bending the torso is often one of folding in the forward direction, 15c. Folding can also occur over other body surfaces. Folding toward the right side is given in 15d, over the back surface in 15e. Other possibilities can occur. The signs are doubled for the greater degree, 15f, 15g.

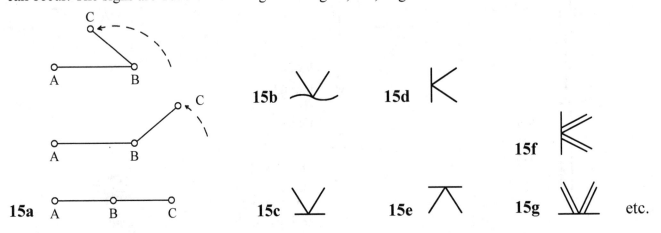

15a

15b

15c

15d

15e

15f

15g   etc.

Unfolding is the reverse of folding. The sign of unfolding, 15h, is the cancellation sign for 'away' with a horizontal line near the bottom. There are no degrees for unfolding, thus only one sign is needed to complete the action. A duration line is attached to indicate timing, 15i. Note the whole torso folding in 15j, and the hand folding and unfolding in 15k.

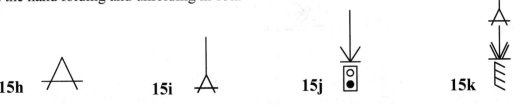

15h

15i

15j

15k

14

SUPPORT, PARTS OF THE BODY

SPRINGING, AERIAL STEPS

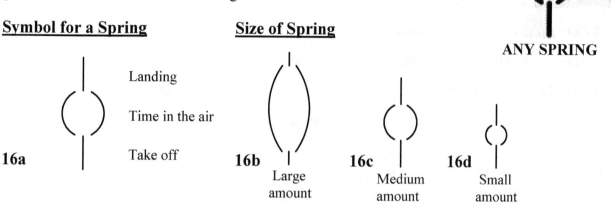

ANY SPRING

All aerial steps, that is, forms of springing, start from a support on the ground,
go into the air and then return to the ground.

Symbol for a Spring   **Size of Spring**

16a Landing

Time in the air

Take off

16b Large amount

16c Medium amount

16d Small amount

Ex. 16b – d illustrates the amount of time spent in the air.

Each form of spring may have a separate start, or they may be rebound, consecutive springs.

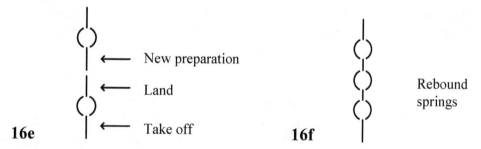

16e ← New preparation
← Land
← Take off

16f Rebound springs

Springs may be linked to travelling:

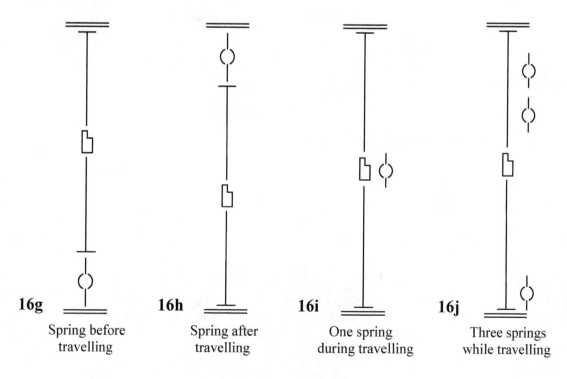

16g Spring before travelling

16h Spring after travelling

16i One spring during travelling

16j Three springs while travelling

15

SPRINGS: THE FIVE BASIC FORMS

There are only five possible springs
using two feet, they are:

Names for Springs

17a	From two feet to two	Jump
17b,c	From one foot to the same	Hop
17d,e	From one foot to the other	Leap
17f,g	From one foot to two	Joining (Ballet term: *Assemblé*)
17h,i	From two feet to one	Separating (Ballet term: *Sissonne*)

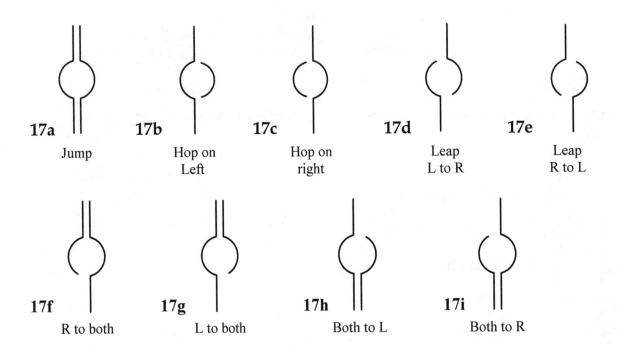

17a	17b	17c	17d	17e
Jump	Hop on Left	Hop on right	Leap L to R	Leap R to L

17f	17g	17h	17i
R to both	L to both	Both to L	Both to R

Combined with Direction

To become more specific, a direction symbol may be added:

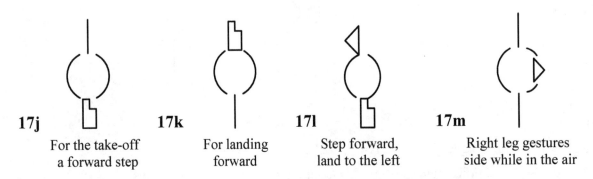

17j	17k	17l	17m
For the take-off a forward step	For landing forward	Step forward, land to the left	Right leg gestures side while in the air

PARTS OF THE BODY

To provide open choice, the sign of 18a, meaning any body part is a combination of the sign for an area and that for a limb. Moving from the general to the specific, the next stage is to indicate the main parts of the body – the areas, the joints, and the limbs.

18a Any body area or limb   **18b** An area   **18c** A limb

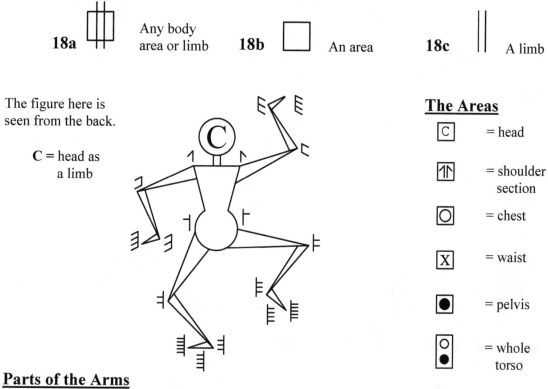

The figure here is seen from the back.

C = head as a limb

The Areas

C	= head
⇑↑	= shoulder section
O	= chest
X	= waist
●	= pelvis
○●	= whole torso

Parts of the Arms

Whole arm	Left		Right		Both	
		Shoulder				Shoulders
Left Right		Elbow				Elbows
		Wrist				Wrists
Both		Hand				Hands
		Fingers				Fingers

Parts of the Legs

Whole leg	Left		Right		Both	
		Hip				Hips
Left Right		Knee				Knees
		Ankle				Ankles
Both		Foot				Feet
		Toes				Toes

CHANGE OF SUPPORT

An angular horizontal line indicates supporting, taking weight.

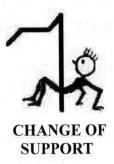

**CHANGE OF
SUPPORT**

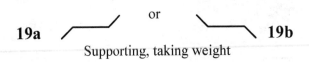

19a   or   19b

Supporting, taking weight

The top end of the line indicates the part that is being supported, the bottom end is the supporting part, often the floor. The duration of the change to a new support is shown by the length of the action which leads to the new support.

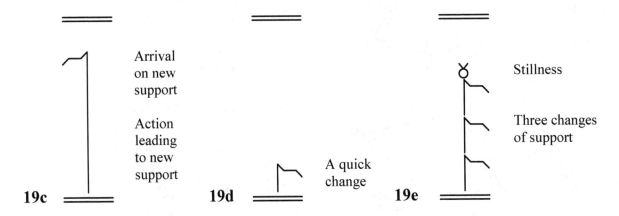

19c — Arrival on new support

Action leading to new support

19d — A quick change

19e — Stillness

Three changes of support

The following indicate what part of the body is being supported.

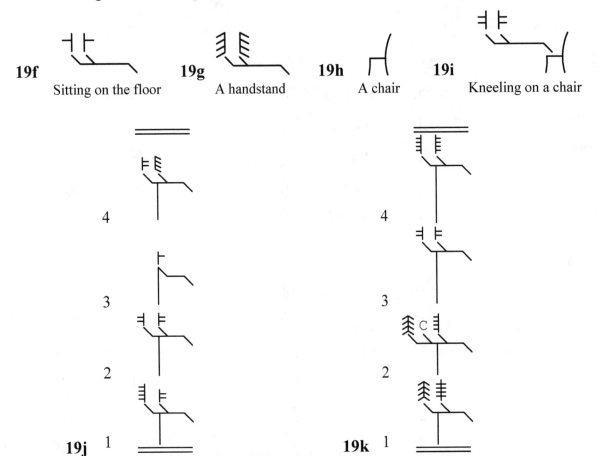

19f Sitting on the floor   **19g** A handstand   **19h** A chair   **19i** Kneeling on a chair

19j   4   3   2   1

19k   4   3   2   1

18

Lying on Different Parts of the Torso

Lying on the front, the back, or on one side is indicated by attaching a small 'tick' to the appropriate side of the torso sign. If no tick is indicated, as in 20a, then on which surface one is lying is not important, it is open to choice.

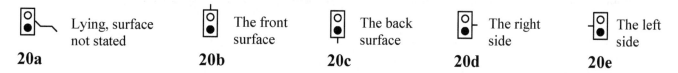

Rolling on the Floor

Rolling on the floor, as in log rolling, is shown by attaching two abbreviated angular supporting lines to the turn symbol to show consecutive supporting. These may be placed on either side, as in 20f, 20g.

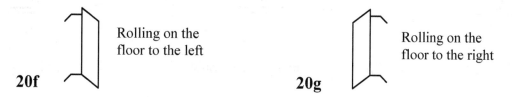

In the following study, changes in supporting on one or another surface of the torso are achieved through rolling.

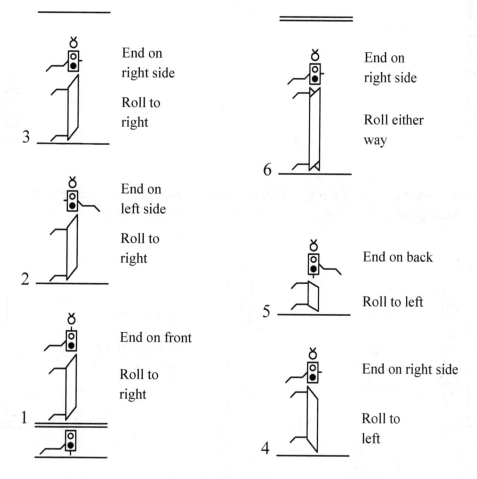

PART LEADING, INITIATING

A movement may be initiated by a particular body part, or that part may lead for the duration of the movement. The symbol for the body part involved is placed within a curved vertical bow next to the movement indication. The length of this bow shows the duration of the leading activity.

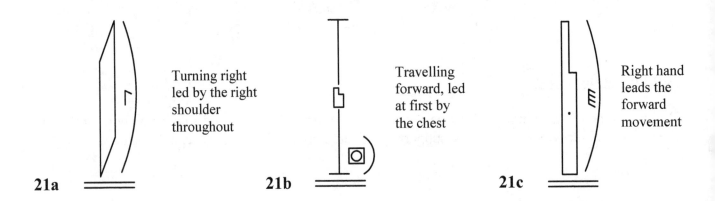

21a   Turning right led by the right shoulder throughout

21b   Travelling forward, led at first by the chest

21c   Right hand leads the forward movement

For left side parts of the body, the bow is usually placed on the left, as an aid in reading.

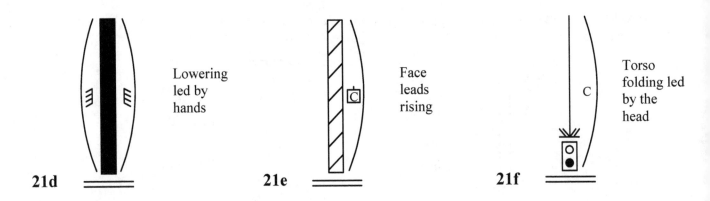

21d   Lowering led by hands

21e   Face leads rising

21f   Torso folding led by the head

There can be a change in part-leading within one movement. This can occur without a pause. At the end of a part leading indication, that part will return to its normal alignment.

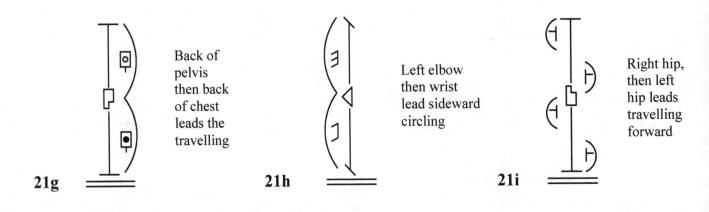

21g   Back of pelvis then back of chest leads the travelling

21h   Left elbow then wrist lead sideward circling

21i   Right hip, then left hip leads travelling forward

CENTER OF GRAVITY

BALANCE

In daily life no thought is given to being in balance, it is expected, but in dance focus on weight placement, centred balance and shifting the weight may be important. Ex. 22a is the sign for the centre of gravity (centre of weight), the point of balance in the body. When the centre of weight is on the vertical line, it is in balance.

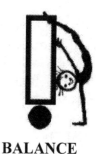

BALANCE

22a Centre of weight centre of gravity)

22b Centre of weight on the vertical line – in balance

Shifting Weight

The minor movement of shifting the weight while still in balance is shown by using straight pins ('tacks'), the point of the pin indicating the direction of the shift. Ex. 22d ends with weight centred.

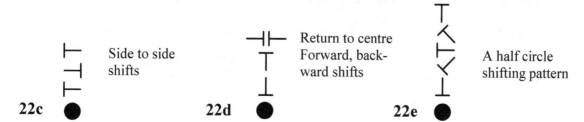

22c Side to side shifts

22d Return to centre Forward, backward shifts

22e A half circle shifting pattern

Centre of Weight Leading

When the centre of weight leads into a direction, for instance, leading into a step, a slight loss of balance occurs. Such leading is indicated by placing the centre of weight sign within the vertical bow.

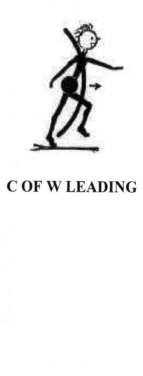

C OF W LEADING

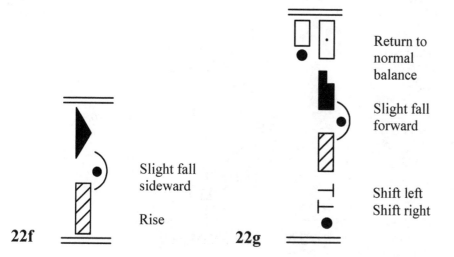

Return to normal balance

Slight fall forward

Shift left Shift right

22f Slight fall sideward

Rise

22g

TRUE FALL

A real, total loss of balance produces the uncomfortable state of falling, total uncontrolled loss of balance. Ex. 22h shows the basic sign for falling, loss of balance, the line through it stating not in balance. The direction of falling is shown by an empty direction symbol; 22i states falling forward, while 22j is falling to the right.

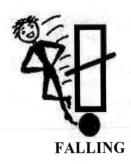

FALLING

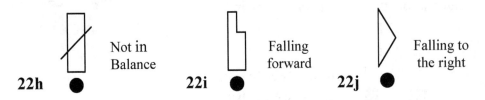

22h — Not in Balance

22i — Falling forward

22j — Falling to the right

Central Fall

A familiar swift lowering to the floor, comparable to a wave breaking on the shore, is often called a 'fall', although the unpleasant experience of true loss of balance does not occur. Such falls can be done in slow motion because at each moment the centre of weight is over a point of support. For this reason they are called "central falls". A vertical arrow pointing downward conveys this idea.

22k — A central fall, any direction

22l — A central fall sideward

22m — A central fall backward

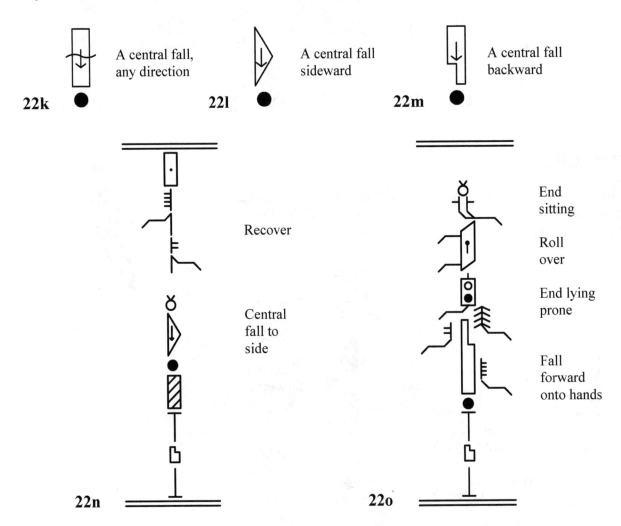

Recover

Central fall to side

22n

End sitting

Roll over

End lying prone

Fall forward onto hands

22o

MOVEMENT INTENTION

TOWARD & AWAY

Movement may be toward a person, an object, a part of the room, or a state of some kind. The symbol of 23a indicates movement toward something, the ad lib. sign provides the open statement.

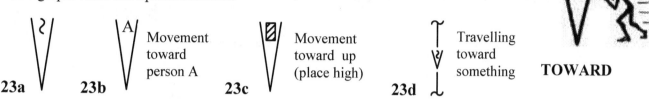

23a Movement **23b** Movement toward person A **23c** Movement toward up (place high) **23d** Travelling toward something **TOWARD**

Movement away is the reverse of movement toward.

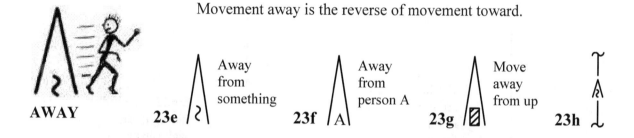

AWAY **23e** Away from something **23f** Away from person A **23g** Move away from up **23h**

DESTINATION, ARRIVE

A movement arriving at a destination is shown by linking the movement indication to the statement of the destination. Ex. 23i shows arrival of some kind. In 23j, the movement ends in a shape. Ex. 23k shows that the path ends at the chair.

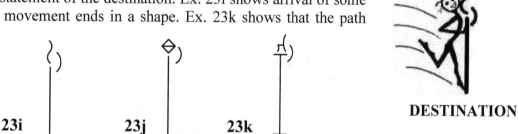

23i **23j** **23k** **DESTINATION**

Location, Parts of the Room

As explained earlier, a square represents an area. By darkening the appropriate part, a particular part of the room can be shown. Ex. 23l shows the main parts of the room or stage. Circling, ending in the centre of the room is given in 23v.

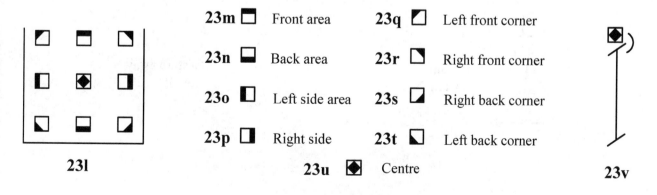

23l

23m ▭ Front area	**23q** ◸ Left front corner	
23n ▭ Back area	**23r** ◹ Right front corner	
23o ▯ Left side area	**23s** ◿ Right back corner	
23p ▮ Right side	**23t** ◺ Left back corner	
	23u ◈ Centre	

23v

TOWARD, AWAY, ARRIVAL

In the following reading sequence 'P' represents a partner.

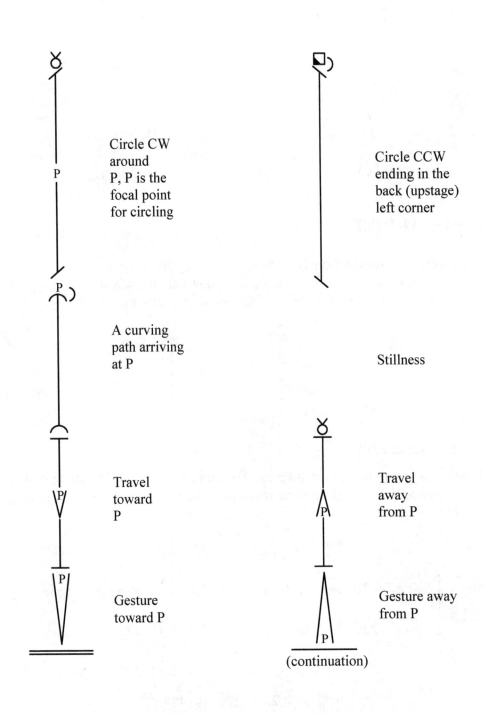

Circle CW around P, P is the focal point for circling

Circle CCW ending in the back (upstage) left corner

A curving path arriving at P

Stillness

Travel toward P

Travel away from P

Gesture toward P

Gesture away from P

(continuation)

RELATIONSHIPS

FORMS OF RELATING

Many movements have as their aim establishing some kind of a relationship to a person, object or part of the room (stage). This relationship is often more important than the kind of movement which produced it. Before specifying a particular form of relationship, the general statement can be made. Ex. 24a is the sign for 'any form of relating'.

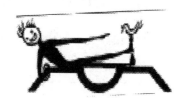

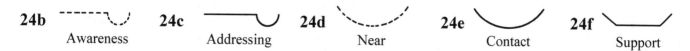

24a　Any form of relating

Different horizontal 'bows' show the different possibilities for relating:

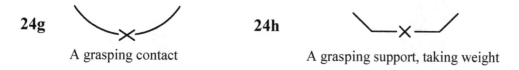

24b Awareness　**24c** Addressing　**24d** Near　**24e** Contact　**24f** Support

Contact, touch may occur with a closing in, a grasping of the object. Similarly, supporting, carrying may also occur with a grasp. To show this, the flexion sign: X is added to the bow, as in 24g and 24h.

24g　A grasping contact　　**24h**　A grasping support, taking weight

The angular support bow of 24f, may also be drawn as 24i or 24j, the lower end represents the floor (when nothing other is stated). The upper end indicates the object, person or body part being supported.

24i　　**24j**

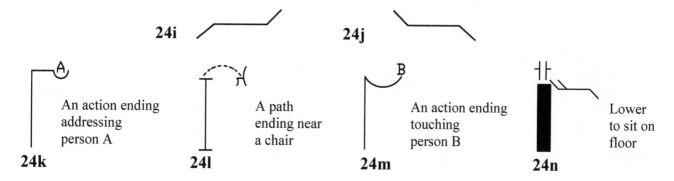

24k An action ending addressing person A

24l A path ending near a chair

24m An action ending touching person B

24n Lower to sit on floor

Retention of a Relationship

If a form of relationship is to be retained, held, the retention sign, 24o, is placed above the horizontal bow. This statement has then to be cancelled. The sign for letting go, releasing a contact, grasp, etc. is shown by the release sign, 24p, which may be drawn horizontally or vertically.

24o Hold　　　　**24p** Release

Reading Sequence

RELATIONSHIPS, DIFFERENT FORMS

The length of the action stroke or other movement symbol indicates how long it takes to achieve the stated relationship.

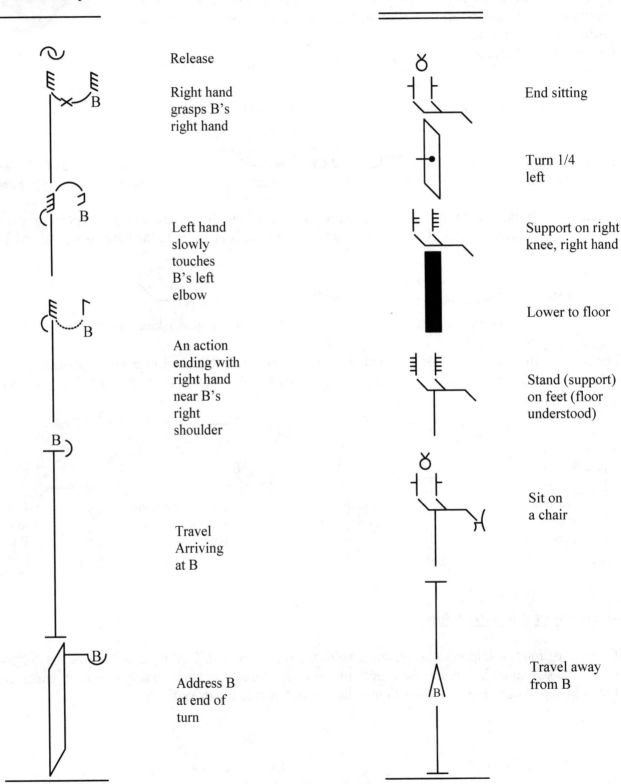

Release

Right hand grasps B's right hand

Left hand slowly touches B's left elbow

An action ending with right hand near B's right shoulder

Travel Arriving at B

Address B at end of turn

End sitting

Turn 1/4 left

Support on right knee, right hand

Lower to floor

Stand (support) on feet (floor understood)

Sit on a chair

Travel away from B

SUPPORTS – STEPS

Because supports are so often on the feet, special shorthand signs have been devised for such steps. Ex. 25a is the indication for supporting on both feet, 25b shows a step on the left foot, with 25c a step on to the right foot. These support indications can be attached to direction symbols to indicate the direction and level for each step. Ex. 25d shows a middle level step forward on the right foot while 25e is a low backward step. Ex. 25f shows stepping to the left side in high level, while 25g is both feet together in place in low level.

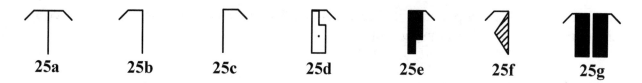

The following reading examples show A: steps in any direction, any level in different timing. B: circling with quick steps then a change of level to a low step. C: direction and levels are shown for this box waltz pattern which concludes with a springing pattern.

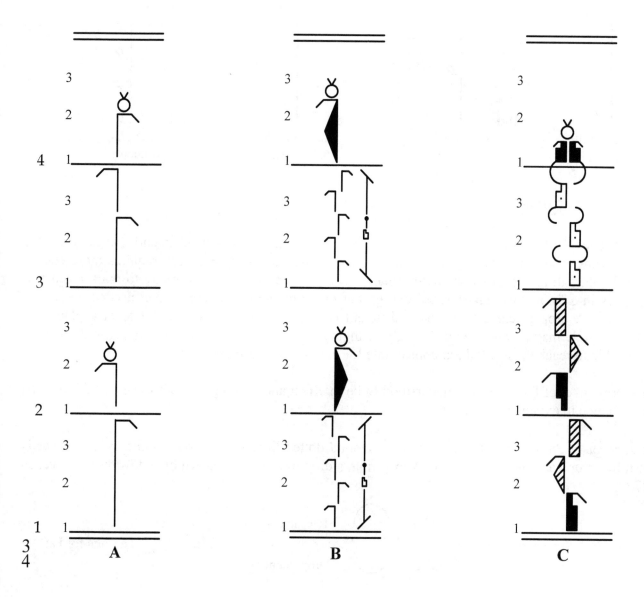

DYNAMICS

The ebb and flow of energy in the body affects the quality and impact of a movement. The interplay of tension and relaxation within the muscles, the increase in force and the letting go, provide a range of movement 'colouring'. How and why these changes take place may rest on many factors. Let us start with the simplest.

Accented Movements

A momentary increase in energy produces an accent, giving that moment more importance. An accent may be slight or may be marked, a strong accent.

A single accent may occur at the start of a movement, in the middle, or at the end. More than one accent may occur during a single movement.

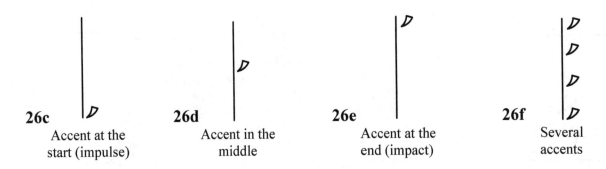

The Concept of 'Par'

Par is that level of energy needed to accomplish a particular movement efficiently without wasted effort or using insufficient energy to function satisfactorily. Jumping naturally requires more energy than walking, sitting requires less energy than standing. Stamping, for example, to mark a musical rhythm, as in a folk dance, takes added energy but may involve more energy than needed, i.e. a rise above Par. A drop in energy may have different causes, different reasons for it to take place. A carefree attitude may produce relaxed, freely swinging movements, or tiredness may cause the person to be unable to reach the level of Par appropriate for the movement in question.

The energy level of Par is usually understood to be in effect and nothing, therefore, needs be indicated until a change in dynamics occurs.

The concept of Par can be illustrated by a horizontal dotted line, 27a. A rise in energy above Par is shown by an upward curve, as in 27b. A lowering, a drop in energy is shown by a downward curve, as in 27c.

27b ⌒ Rise in energy

27a Par: - - - - - - - - - - - 　 - - - - - - 　 27d ⋈ The sign for Par

27c ⌣ Drop in energy

Only general statements are given for the degree of rise or drop in energy; a white circle for a slight degree, a black circle for a marked degree. These are placed on the appropriate curved bow.

Degree of Rise or Lowering of Energy

The following illustrate two degrees in rise above Par and two below Par.

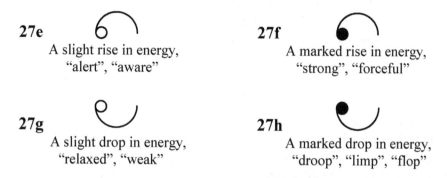

27e   A slight rise in energy, "alert", "aware"

27f   A marked rise in energy, "strong", "forceful"

27g   A slight drop in energy, "relaxed", "weak"

27h   A marked drop in energy, "droop", "limp", "flop"

These symbols are placed next to the movement indication they qualify.

Relation to Gravity

The pull of gravity is with us all the time. In our Par relation to gravity, we use the amount of energy needed for our daily tasks. We may give in to gravity, that is, allow gravity to take over when relaxing, through tiredness, or when fainting, the extreme case in which all muscular tension lets go. We fight gravity in lifting objects, in lifting ourselves when we climb stairs, or when jumping, springing high off the ground.

The vertical line of gravity is visualised as an imaginary line centred on the upward or downward bow.

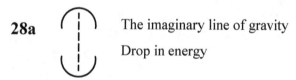

28a   The imaginary line of gravity

Drop in energy

To indicate a rise or drop of energy in relation to gravity, the white or black circle is centred in the curved bow on the imagined line of gravity.

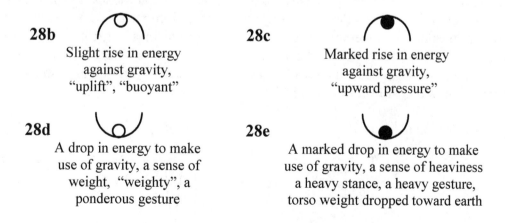

28b   Slight rise in energy against gravity, "uplift", "buoyant"

28c   Marked rise in energy against gravity, "upward pressure"

28d   A drop in energy to make use of gravity, a sense of weight, "weighty", a ponderous gesture

28e   A marked drop in energy to make use of gravity, a sense of heaviness a heavy stance, a heavy gesture, torso weight dropped toward earth

How we make use of gravity in movement can be considered in four categories: 1) practical, functional need; 2) the result of an emotional state; 3) the need for a physical sense of body mass; 4) the production of sound, as in clapping or stamping a rhythm.

Timing, Duration of Dynamic Indications

A dynamic marking can be indicated at the point in an action when that quality occurs. This could be at the beginning, in the middle, or at the end, as illustrated in 29a-c.

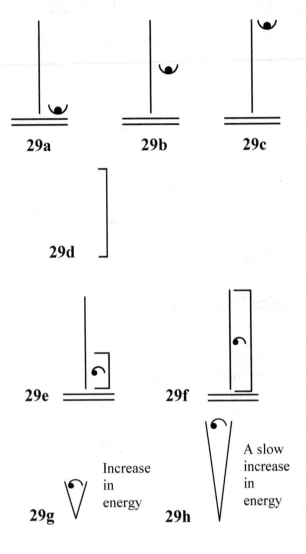

Additional information is often placed in an angular vertical bracket, 29d, placed alongside the movement(s) to which the information belongs. For dynamics, this angular bracket refers to a physical use of energy or a lack of it.

The duration of a dynamic indication, which is, how long a dynamic quality is maintained is shown by the length of the vertical bracket in which it is placed. Within this bracket the stated dynamic will be constant. In 29e, a brief duration is shown; in 29f, it is maintained for a longer time.

When an increase or decrease sign is used, the length of that sign indicates how long the stated quality should grow or diminish, i.e. become established or fade away. Ex. 29g shows a short duration; in 29h, it takes quite a bit longer.

Cancellation

When no dynamic indication is given, the performance is expected to be at the level of Par appropriate for that particular kind of action. Cancellation of a dynamic indication occurs when another dynamic aspect is indicated, as in 30a. A movement that follows a statement in a vertical bracket, 30b, will return to neutral, that is, an unstated Par is understood. However, when a direct statement is needed, the symbol for Par can be used to indicate a return to that state. In 30c a return to Par is shown to occur quickly. The return to Par is of a slower duration in 30d.

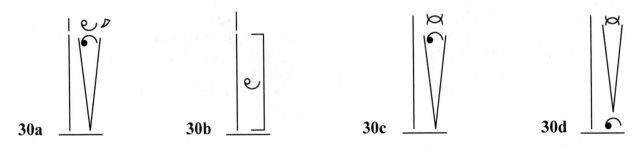

NOTES

NOTES

NOTES

NOTES

NOTES

NOTES

NOTES

CPSIA information can be obtained
at www.ICGtesting.com
Printed in the USA
LVHW051542150721
692810LV00008B/492

9 780955 430503